BASICS OF WIRE AND CATHETER BASED PROCEDURES

FOR

Beginners And Peri-Procedure Personnel

FIRST EDITION

ISIBOR ARHUIDESE, MD MPH

International Standard Book Number: 978-1-7363767-1-3

Library of Congress Control Number: 2020912648

The author and publishers welcome feedback, questions or comments on the content and application. For comments, questions, sales, bulk purchase, reprint requests or permissions to use material from this book contact: the.endo.book@gmail.com

Notices

Information and best practice in this field are constantly being updated. As experience and research expand our understanding, it may be necessary to implement changes in practice and treatment. Practitioners must rely on their own experience and knowledge. Be mindful of safety of self and others, including those for whom you have a professional responsibility when implementing any of the methods described in this book.

With respect to the devices and products described in the following material, readers are directed to check the most current information provided by the manufacturer of each product. It is advised that you verify the recommended indications, methods of use and contraindications before using any product or treatment.

It is the responsibility of practitioners, relying on their own experience and knowledge of their patients, to make diagnoses, to determine best treatment for each patient, and to take all appropriate precautions with regards to safety.

To the fullest extent permitted by law, the publishers, authors, contributors, and editors do not assume any liability for injury and/or damage to persons or property as a matter of product liability, negligence or otherwise, or from any use or operation of the methods, products, instructions, or ideas contained within the enclosed material.

Dedicated to my parents James and Veronica Arhuidese, for prioritizing discipline and hard work, and for loving, teaching and correcting us in a way that no one else can.

And

To those who understand that the transfer of knowledge or skill can be devoid of humiliation. To the giants upon whose shoulders we stand and to those who inspire us to be giants.

IJA

March 2020

Special thanks to Dr. Murray L. Shames for providing expert review of the contents of this book. As well as to my teachers and the peri-procedure staff who share the science and art of successful procedures with me.

Forward

Dramatic change has occurred in the evolution of minimally invasive therapies in the past four decades. The efficiency and precision required to safely execute these procedures coupled with the flux in personnel and experience raises the need for reference texts for participants at all levels.

Basics of Wire and Catheter Based Procedures for Beginners and Peri-Procedure Personnel fulfills an essential gap in material for teaching and reference for technicians, nurses and other peri-procedural personnel who contribute to the success of these procedures. The content also serves as a valuable primer for trainees who may go on to seek detailed knowledge or skill.

With the aid of diagrams and in a manner that is easy to understand, Dr Arhuidese describes concepts that enhance the safety and success of these minimally invasive procedures to the benefit of patients. This book is a must read for every peri-procedure staff and trainee.

Murray L Shames, MD DFSVS
Professor of Vascular Surgery and Radiology
Chief, Division of Vascular Surgery
University of South Florida, Morsani College of Medicine
President of Association of Program Directors in Vascular Surgery

Table of Contents

Chapter 1

INTRODUCTION

The number and complexity of catheter- based procedures for the diagnosis and treatment of disorders of the cardiovascular system have increased over time. An aging population and advancements in technology suggest that the trend will persist. Accordingly, the number of personnel tasked with performing these procedures is increasing. Inevitably, beginners must learn the craft in order to progress and satisfy the demand. Peri-procedural personnel also need to be familiar with the procedure and devices.

The cardiovascular system is pressurized and fluid-filled. End organs rely on its continuity. As such, wire- and catheter-based procedures must be precise and efficient to minimize adverse events, which can be unforgiving. These procedures involve multiple moving parts that require coordinated teamwork. For the beginner, understanding the components-what to do and what not to do- can be challenging. Indeed, the learning curve is steep and laden with anxiety. Procedures that involve wire- and catheter- based traversal of the cardiovascular system are commonly performed in the endovascular, interventional cardiology, or interventional radiology domains. There is a paucity of reference texts as well as variability in the early learning experience for beginners and personnel who may be tasked with assisting with device retrieval, preparation, exchange, or other parts of the procedure. Yet, their actions or inactions weigh immensely on the safety, efficiency, and success of the procedure.

This book provides a concise introduction to the wire- and catheter- based procedures of the cardiovascular system. It describes the general concepts as well as some of the commonly used equipment and tools. A good grasp of the content prepares the reader for practical learning and facilitates rapid ascent of the learning curve. Experience has shown that personnel who understand why things are being done are better positioned to anticipate and prepare for potential next steps, to adapt when the tempo or objectives change, and ultimately to play their role in the execution of a safe and successful procedure.

Chapter 2

LOCATION, PERSONNEL, AND EQUIPMENT

Wire- and catheter- based procedures that involve access and traversal of the vascular system are performed in the following settings:

- The endovascular, interventional cardiology, or interventional radiology suite
- The operating room
- The hybrid operating room

Some degree of overlap exists because these locations support the resources necessary for safe and efficient traversal of the cardiovascular system, however, each has unique characteristics.

Endovascular, Interventional Radiology, or Cardiology Suite

This suite supports needle-based (percutaneous) access of the vascular system without the need for a formal incision or "cut down." These rooms also support interventional radiology procedures that may or may not involve planned entry into the vascular system. When referred to as the interventional cardiology suite- or more commonly the "cath lab"- the suite is tailored to support heart catheterization and other minimally invasive cardiac procedures. The endovascular, interventional radiology, or cardiology suite may be located in an office-based lab, ambulatory surgery center, or in-hospital setting. Most of the procedures performed in these locations are executed without the need for general anesthesia. However, it can be delivered if necessary.

Operating Room

The operating room is the traditional location for procedures that involve an incision and can support deep forms of anesthesia. Mobile equipment such as the portable fluoroscopy machine (C-arm) and fluoroscopy-compatible table allow execution of endovascular procedures in the operating room. The procedures performed in this location can be exclusively wire- and catheter- based or they may be adjuncts to open surgery.

Hybrid Operating and Minimally Invasive Suite

The complexity of endovascular and minimally invasive cardiac procedures has increased over time. The hybrid suite evolved to satisfy the ergonomic needs of these procedures.

4

Several conditions that were previously treated only with open surgery now have wire- and catheter-based alternatives for treatment. In some instances, the risk of conversion to open surgery is high, hence the need to perform the minimally invasive alternative in an environment that can support open surgery if the situation arises. The hybrid suite is so named because it has full operating room and endovascular procedure capabilities. The ergonomic and safety modifications deployed in hybrid suites include its large size, mounted fluoroscopy units, monitors optimized in size and image quality, fluoroscopy tables with controls that are accessible to the operator, adjoining control/viewing room with audio-visual connections, and the myriad of fixed and mobile protections from radiation.

Personnel

The personnel involved in these procedures depend on the type and complexity of the procedure. These include a combination and number of:

- Operators-surgeons, cardiologists, radiologists
- Radiology technicians
- Surgical technicians
- Nurses
- Anesthesia providers

- Trainees

Equipment

Some of the common equipment, devices, and supplies are listed below. This list is in no way exhaustive.

- Imaging equipment: Fluoroscopy machine and monitors, conventional ultrasound, intravascular ultrasound, computed tomography fusion technology and display, optical coherence tomography, near infra-red spectroscopy
- Support surfaces: Procedure table, back table, and extensions
- Anesthesia and patient-monitoring equipment, monitors, and medications
- Radiation safety shields
- Access/navigational tools: Needles, wires, catheters, sheaths
- Intervention devices: Balloons, stents, stent grafts (endografts), and an inexhaustible list of specialty tools and devices
- Access closure devices
- Supplies: Sterile gowns, gloves, gauze, surgical blades, suture, clamps, needle drivers, etc.

- Solutions and medications: Saline, contrast, heparin, or other anticoagulant alternatives

Chapter 3

RADIATION AND RADIATION SAFETY

Radiation is harnessed in medicine for diagnostic and therapeutic purposes. It can be used to visualize anatomic depths that cannot be seen from the surface. Ionizing radiation in the form of X-rays is invisible. The effects are potent and can be seen in a variety of output modalities such as plain X-ray films, computed tomography scans, or fluoroscopy monitors. Despite the wide range of diagnostic and therapeutic application of radiation, it has undesirable side effects. These include:

- Rash
- Hair loss
- Burns
- Ulcers
- Cataracts
- Cancer
- Infertility
- Fetal abnormalities

Repeated exposure to radiation places patients and personnel at high risk of adverse events, hence the need to balance diagnostic/therapeutic use with associated risk. Although the

9

effects of radiation can be seen on monitors, the spectrum of radiation used is not directly visible. In addition, the aforementioned adverse effects of radiation on humans are often distant from the source in time and space. These subtle yet deleterious effects of medical grade radiation must be acknowledged, and meticulous steps should be taken to prevent them. An understanding of how X-rays work in the procedure suite is a key aspect of risk reduction.

Radiation Emission and Image Acquisition

In fluoroscopy, radiation in the form of X-rays is applied in a static, pulsed, or continuous manner to visualize anatomy in real time. The radiation source and detection system (fluoroscopy machine) is designed to allow its movement around the patient in order to image selected body segments from a variety of angles. The fluoroscopy machines are commonly seen as portable units (C -arm) or ceiling/floor mounted units.

X-rays are emitted from a medical grade radioactive source within the fluoroscopy machine. They pass through the radiolucent table, then through the patient's body, and is absorbed by the detector/image intensifier. These absorbed rays are then transduced into an image and displayed on a monitor (figure 3.1). Several characteristics of the X-ray beam such as the intensity, area of exposure, duration of exposure, magnification, continuity, and interaction with contrast media can be manipulated by the operator.

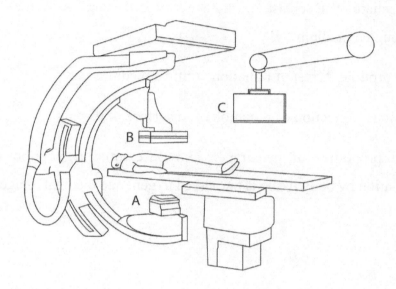

Figure 3.1 Fluoroscopy machine. A: radiation source; B: Image intensifier; C: monitor

Penetrance, Attenuation, Absorption, and Scatter

Penetrance, attenuation, absorption, and scatter are pertinent properties of radiation used in medicine (figure 3.2).

Penetrance: Ability of radiation to pass through a medium in its path

Attenuation: Decrease in potency of radiation as it travels through a medium

Absorption: Arrest of radiation within a medium

Scatter: Reflection of radiation off a surface in its path

The properties of penetrance and differential absorption of radiation by body tissue is harnessed to generate medical images.

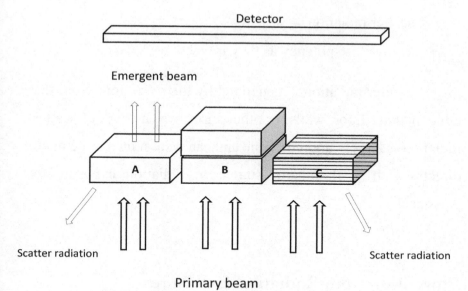

Figure 3.2: Penetrance, attenuation. absorption and scatter

A: Penetrance through the medium with attenuation of emergent beam
B: Arrest of radiation due to thickness of medium
C: Arrest of radiation due to density of medium

The following events occur when the X-ray beam is directed at the specific location on the patient:

- Some X-rays pass through the table and the patient and are absorbed by the detector.
- Some X-rays are absorbed by the table and patient.

13

- Some X-rays are reflected off the table and patient, i.e., scatter radiation.
- X-rays lose potency as they travel over distance.

Scatter radiation is generated by the reflections from the table, patient, floor, walls, or other surfaces. The path of scatter radiation is largely unpredictable and can be assumed to be in all directions. It is the major source of radiation exposure to personnel.

Prevention from Radiation Exposure

The properties of X-ray absorption by dense media and loss of potency over distance are harnessed for personnel protection. Despite the exposure to scatter radiation, it is known that individual risk is minimized when precautionary measures are deployed. The first line of defense against radiation exposure is to avoid it. Therefore, only personnel who are essential to achieving procedural or educational goals should be in the room. Persons who may be interested in the procedure but not directly involved are encouraged to stay in adjoining rooms where available. These rooms typically have transparent, radio-protective screens and audiovisual connections for communication.

It is mandatory for in-room personnel to wear radio-protective gear. Lead is the most common dense material used to minimize radiation exposure; it decreases radiation exposure by absorption. Some personal protective gear and shields are listed below:

- Lead-impregnated apparel covering the torso and lower extremities circumferentially at least to the knee (figure 3.3). Lead content should be 1mm thickness for pregnant personnel and 0.5mm thickness for all others.
- Thyroid shield
- Eye covering

Appropriate storage of the apparel is key to preventing mechanical disruption of the lead content and loss of protective properties (figure 3.4). Other protective shields may be fixed or mobile and can be positioned around the patient, personnel, or equipment (figure 3.5). Examples are:

- Table mounted shields/skirts
- Ceiling mounted shields
- Mobile barrier shields

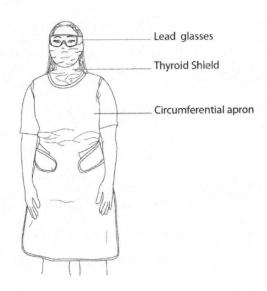

Figure 3.3 Lead apparel

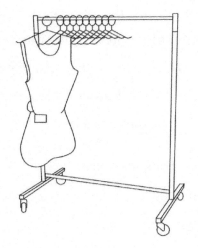

Figure 3.4 Storage for lead apparel

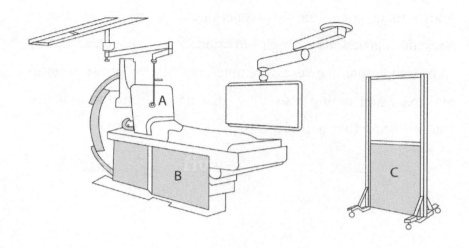

Figure 3.5 Radiation shields mounted from the ceiling (A); procedure table (B); and a mobile shield (C)

The potency of radiation as it travels through a medium is governed by the inverse square law. According to this law, the intensity of radiation changes by the square of the change in distance from the source. For example, decreasing the distance from the radiation source by a factor of 3 decreases the intensity of the radiation at the new location by a factor of 9. When the distance is increased by a factor of 5 the intensity of radiation decreases by a factor of 25 and so forth (figure 3.6). Accordingly, maintaining a distance from the fluoroscopy machine is an effective way of decreasing radiation exposure. It is recommended that personnel stay at the furthest distance that allows them to execute their function and to take several steps back during periods of high radiation emission such as during fluoroscopy runs. The use of remote-controlled contrast injectors and extension tubing also allow distancing from the radiation source during fluoroscopic runs.

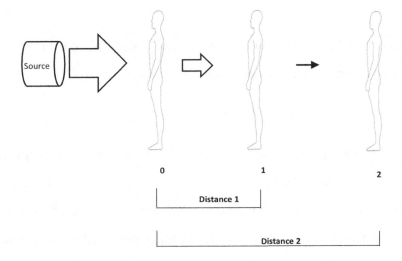

Figure 3.6 Radiation exposure decreases with increase in distance from source. Intensity (I-1) at point 1 is equal to intensity (I-0) at point 0 divided by (distance 1)^2. Intensity (I-2) at point 2 is equal to intensity (I-0) at point 0 divided by (distance 2)^2

The term "As Low as Reasonably Achievable" (ALARA) refers to principles that allow the use of radiation to achieve diagnostic or therapeutic goals while minimizing exposure and risk to patients and team members. Operator-dependent maneuvers such as collimation of the radiation beam, adjustment of the relative height of the procedure table/patient, X-ray source and detector, type and duration of fluoroscopic runs, frame rates, and gantry angles can be modified to satisfy the principles of ALARA. It is also good practice for the operator to ensure that all personnel have protective gear and equipment in place before radiation is activated. Pre-procedure planning and communication can minimize the need for multiple images. A culture in which all personnel are aware, and in which they individually and collectively take steps to mitigate radiation exposure, is ideal. It is important to ensure that the fluoroscopy machine is inactivated when not in use to avoid accidental trigger by unsuspecting staff. Cleaning and custodial personnel who may not be aware of the accidental emissions and may not be wearing protective gear are particularly prone to exposure in this manner. However, anyone can be affected. It is recommended that personnel speak up when a component of radiation protection is not being applied and action is taken to re-instate it.

Monitoring

Radiation monitoring ensures that exposure remains within safe limits and appropriate action is taken when significant events occur. Elements of radiation monitoring include:

- Measurement and documentation of the amount of radiation utilized for each procedure.

- All personnel wear a radiation monitoring badge outside of their lead apparel to monitor individual exposure over time. Pregnant personnel should wear two badges: the regular badge outside the lead apparel and another one inside (fetal monitor).

- Most institutions have radiation safety officers who periodically inspect radiation equipment, protective gear, and personnel exposure levels. None the less, radiation safety is everyone's responsibility. It is important to know the institution's radiation safety officer and policies.

Chapter 4

PROCEDURE SETUP

Planning and organization are key aspects of wire- and catheter-based interventions. The patient is at the center of the procedure. The arrangement of personnel and equipment positioned around the patient can make for a smooth procedure or it could be a recipe for chaos and errors.

The Patient

The following steps are useful in preparing the patient for the procedure:

- Confirm the patient's identity upon arrival in the procedure room.
- Ensure the patient is placed on the appropriate procedure table (see section on procedure tables).
- Transfer the patient to the procedure table with caution and appropriate assistance to minimize fall risk.
- Place appropriate restraints and extensions.
- Determine the type of intravenous access, hemodynamic monitoring, and approach to urinary bladder emptying necessary for the procedure.
- Adjust patient position in line with procedural objectives.

21

- Determine the minimum amount of body exposure required to perform the procedure.

- Communicate the purpose of exposing the body part to the patient.

- Expose the part of the body necessary for the procedure while also taking steps to protect patient privacy.

- Clip excess hair at the access site. Exercise caution to avoid skin injuries as this is a common source of pain and discomfort, especially after application of skin preparation agents.

- Shield any orifice that is close to the access site and is capable of yielding effluents that might contaminate the site. These may include the perineum, colostomy, urostomy, and tracheostomy.

- Pay attention to body habitus and special needs. For example, bariatric patients might require adjunct maneuvers such as elevation of the pannus to expose a femoral access site.

- Apply sterile preparation agents.

- Apply sterile drapes.

Procedure Table

The procedure table supports the patient during the procedure. It is radiolucent to allow passage of X-rays. The table can be manipulated during the procedure to adjust the position of the patient relative to the equipment. The following are relevant aspects of the procedure table to note:

- Ensure it is radiolucent (compatible with fluoroscopy) because not all procedure tables are radiolucent. This is important in locations where the table may not be fixed such as in the operating room.

- With the part of the body to be imaged borne in mind, orient the table such that its base allows for easy movement of the x-ray machine around the area of interest. For example, if the area of interest is in the upper body (neck/chest), the table should be positioned such that the base is under the legs. Conversely, if the lower extremity is the area of interest, then the base should be positioned under the upper body (figure 4.1).

- Ensure that the height and inclination can be adjusted.

- Ensure that it can support the patient's weight. Bariatric patients might require special tables to support their weight. Know the table weight limits in your institution and how to get special tables if necessary.

- Place the table in the center of the room or appropriate location with ample space on all sides for equipment and personnel. It may be necessary to position the table, access site, or target location equidistant between ceiling mounted lights. This is important in the operating/hybrid rooms where lighting is crucial in visualizing incised body segments/cavities.
- Determine if the patient's height, or length of tools/devices warrant table extensions.

The position of table extensions and other equipment should allow the movement of the fluoroscopy machine around the patient. The position and path of the fluoroscopy machine is influenced by the access site and the body area of interest. Communication with the operator is crucial in this regard.

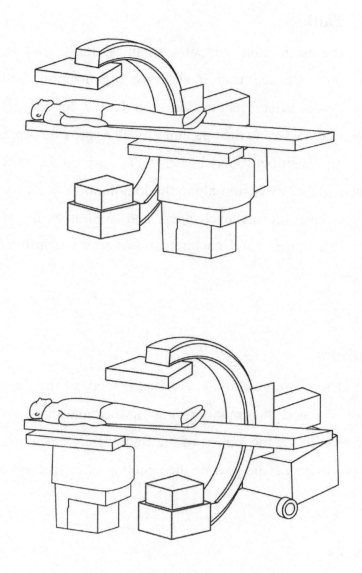

Figure 4.1 Orient the table and its base in a manner that allows the X-ray machine to be maneuvered around the area of interest on the patient.

Back Table

The back table supports supplies, tools, and devices during and between use. Back table organization facilitates efficiency and safety. Its position should allow for easy transfer of tools and devices to the operator as well as provide support for devices in transition. It may be helpful to position the back table or place a table extension-along the longitudinal axis of access. This facilitates device exchanges, and minimizes the risk of device dislodgment and contamination under the influence of gravity.

Monitors

The monitors provide a visual display of the radiologic results. Position the monitor(s) at a location that does not interfere with the movement of the fluoroscopy machine and at an appropriate distance within the operator's line of sight.

Devices

The list of tools, devices, and supplies used in these procedures is vast and it continues to expand with new technology. The devices utilized for a procedure depend on the objective. Accordingly, it is important to know the following:

- The objective of the procedure
- The basic equipment/tools necessary to start the procedure
- The equipment/tools that may be required as the procedure progresses. These may be placed within easy reach but not opened.
- The location for all other devices and the backup storage locations

It may be useful to have carts that contain commonly used tools/devices. These carts can be brought within or close to the procedure room for easy retrieval. Well organized and labeled shelves also facilitate efficient device retrieval. It is good practice to notify personnel responsible for restocking the shelves when persons pulling supplies for a procedure notice any depletion in stock. This provides another line of defense against lack of access to devices when they are needed. Over time and with experience, personnel gain a better grasp of what is needed for every procedure and operator specific preferences. Written notes of basic tools and operator's preferences are helpful. It is recommended that personnel communicate robustly in order to facilitate adequate preparation and to avoid wasteful retrieval of devices that may not be used.

Lighting

The lights in the room may be modified to suit the type and stage of the procedure. In some instances, the lights are dimmed to provide visual contrast on the monitors, while in others, the lights may be turned up to the maximum. It is important to know:

- The location of all light controls
- How to select specific lights or modify their intensity

Chapter 5

DEVICES AND DEVICE PREPARATION

The cardiovascular system has a tree-like design of vessels that convey blood from the heart to the rest of the body and vice versa. During the procedure, vascular access is obtained at one location and the vascular tree is traversed to reach the target area for diagnosis or therapeutic intervention. Accordingly, the tools and devices can be broadly categorized into those used for:

- Access/navigation
- Intervention

There is a wide array of tools, devices, implants, and supplies in use. This chapter provides a description of the common ones and their preparation for use. Further details can be obtained from each manufacturers guide.

It is important to maintain sterility in the retrieval, preparation, and use of every tool or device. Aseptic precautions are crucial to preventing implant, local, remote, or systemic infections. Infections are a major source of morbidity, mortality, and strain on health care resources.

The basic principle of wire- and catheter- based procedures involves sliding one tool/device over or through another. Friction opposes this motion and the resistance to motion is increased by debris on the track such as blood and/or clots. For this reason, a common component of device preparation is flushing or wiping of the track. This minimizes friction by lubrication, clears obstructive debris, and increases efficiency of motion. Plain or heparinized saline is the most common solution applied for this purpose. Special attention should be paid to devices and ports that should not be flushed, and to patients with allergy to heparin.

Access and Navigation

Access and navigation tools are used to access the vessel, secure the access point, and navigate the length, branches, and turns of the vascular tree between the point of access and the target. Collectively, these tools secure access to the target and they include:

- Needles
- Wires
- Catheters
- Sheaths

Needles

Hollow needles are used to gain access to the vascular system. The hollow nature of the needle allows back flow of blood during vessel puncture thus alerting the operator that the needle is in the vessel lumen (figure 5.1). The hollow needle also allows insertion of the wire.

Example needle diameters: 18Ga, 21Ga

In the gauge measurement system, diameter decreases with increasing gauge number. Hence, the 21Ga needle (mini-stick) has a smaller diameter than the 18Ga needle (angio-access). The 21Ga needle will conduct a wire that is 0.018 (0.021) inches or less in diameter. The 18Ga needle will conduct a wire that is 0.035 (0.038) inches or less in diameter.

Preparation

-Flush needles prior to use or reuse to remove any blood clots.

- Safely store needles between use to prevent injury to personnel.

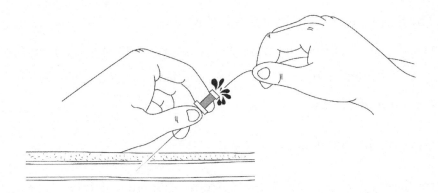

Figure 5.1 Needle access

Wires

A wire is a long, non-hollow cylinder in basic design (figure 5.2). It is steered within the vascular tree to the target. There is a wide spectrum of wire lengths, diameters, strengths, coatings, tip shapes and conformability. Some wires are modular and can be extended. A request for a wire usually involves the type, diameter, and length.

Example wire diameters: 0.010in, 0.014in, 0.016in, 0.018in, 0.035in

Example wire lengths: 40cm, 150cm, 180cm, 260cm, 300cm

The material and coating of a wire determines its handling characteristics. Hydrophilic wires are worthy of special mention because they are slippery to handle. Handling these wires warrants extreme caution to avoid dislodgement from the target, extrusion from the body, or contamination. The pinch/fingertip grip is a good method for handling hydrophilic wires compared to the pulp grip (figure 5.3). It is important to deliver or load the wire with its leading/front end. This end is modified to minimize trauma to the vessel and to satisfy working needs. This end may be softer or have a smoother tip. Between use, the wire may be formed into a coil and placed in a bowl of saline (figure 5.4) or placed in the plastic coil casing (figure 5.2c).

Preparation

-Long wires are often delivered to the back table in a coiled plastic casing (the snail). The casing can be flushed through one of the open ends before the wire is removed (figure 5.5).

-Wipe the wire with a moist piece of gauze after a tool or device traverses it. Extreme caution is warranted during this maneuver to avoid dislodging the wire from its position.

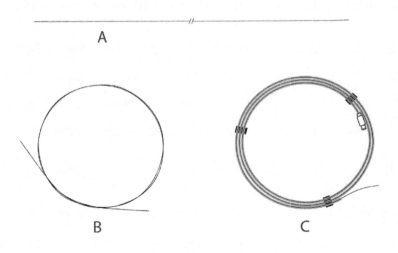

Figure 5.2 Wires. A: straight; B: coiled; C: in its casing

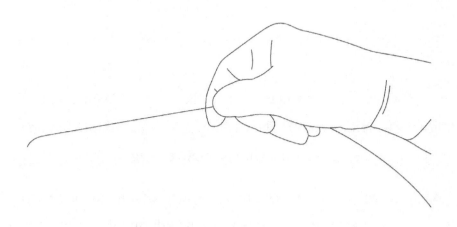

Figure 5.3 Pinch grip

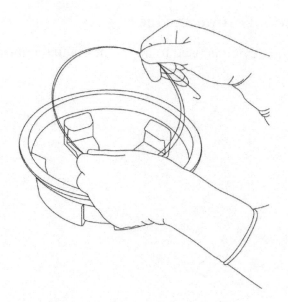

Figure 5.4 Wire storage in bowl of saline

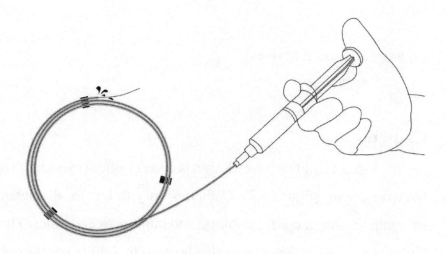

Figure 5.5 Flushing wire casing

Wire adjunct: Torque device

A torque device is used to augment manual control of the wire (figure 5.6).

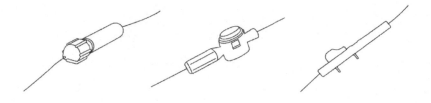

Figure 5.6 Torque devices

Catheter

A catheter in its basic design is a long hollow cylinder that fits over a wire (figure 5.7). Catheters vary in length, diameter, strength, tip shape, conformability, and number of end holes. The hollow nature of catheters can also be used to deliver contrast or medications to the target and to transduce pressure at various locations in the vascular tree. A request for a catheter often includes the type, length, and diameter. The basic properties of the catheter such as the diameter and length may be printed on the external end for reference.

Example catheter lengths: 45cm, 65cm, 90cm, 100cm, 135cm, 150cm

Example catheter diameters: 2.1Fr, 2.3Fr, 2.6Fr, 4Fr, 4.2Fr, 5Fr, 6Fr, 7Fr, 8Fr

Preparation

-Flush catheter before and between use (figure 5.8)

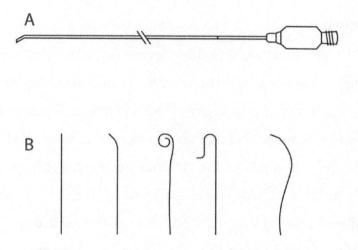

Figure 5.7 A. Catheter and B. Examples of catheter tips

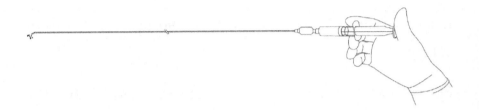

Figure 5.8 Flushing catheter

Sheath

The sheath is a hollow device that is used to secure the point of vascular access (Figure 5.9). It supports navigation to the target and provides a highway across branches and turns that have been crossed so that the maneuvers that were used to cross such difficult points of the vascular tree need not be performed each time a device is transferred to the target site. The cardiovascular system is a pressurized fluid filled system. As such the point of entry into the system must be protected from bleeding. Most sheaths have a one-way valve at the exterior end to allow insertion of tools and devices without bleeding. The valve may be fixed or adjustable.

Sheaths also have a side port to allow for injection of contrast, medications, or saline (figure 5.9A). The side port can also be used to withdraw blood or transduce pressure. The side port can be locked and unlocked for these purposes. The tip of the sheath ends abruptly and is circular in cross section. This tip can cause trauma to the vessel or embolization if the sheath is advanced without its introducer/dilator/stylet (figure 5.10A). To prevent vessel trauma, sheaths are inserted and advanced over a wire with an introducer in its lumen. The introducer tapers the circular tip of the sheath and minimizes the aforementioned risk to the vessel (figure 5.10B). Having the introducer locked in place prior to advancing the sheath is important to ensure that the introducer does not back out of the sheath when the sheath is being advanced.

Sheaths vary in type, length, and diameter. Therefore, a request for a sheath should contain these characteristics. Specialty sheaths that allow adjustment of the shape of the tip also exist. Example sheath diameters: 5Fr, 6Fr, 7Fr, 8Fr, 12Fr, 18Fr

Example sheath lengths: 6cm, 10cm, 45cm, 55cm, 70cm, 90cm

Preparation:

-Flush the sheath before and between use (figure 5.11 A)

-Ensure the side port is locked to the patient before loading onto the wire in order to prevent blood loss after insertion (figure 5.11 B).

-Insert the introducer/dilator/stylet into the sheath and ensure it snaps into place before loading it onto the wire (figure 5.11 C & D).

Maintenance

-Maintain constant flow of saline (drip line) or intermittently flush the sheath through the side port to prevent clot formation within the sheath.

-Pay attention to the location of the sheath to prevent dislodgement especially during device on- or off-loading

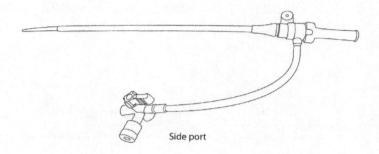

Side port

Figure 5.9 A Sheath with introducer/dilator/stylet inserted

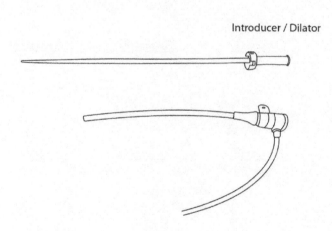

Introducer / Dilator

Figure 5.9 B Sheath separate from introducer/dilator/stylet

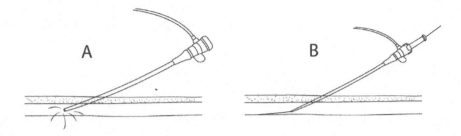

Figure 5.10 A: Advancing a sheath without the introducer causes trauma to the vessel. B: Sheaths should be advanced over a wire with the introducer/dilator/stylet locked into place

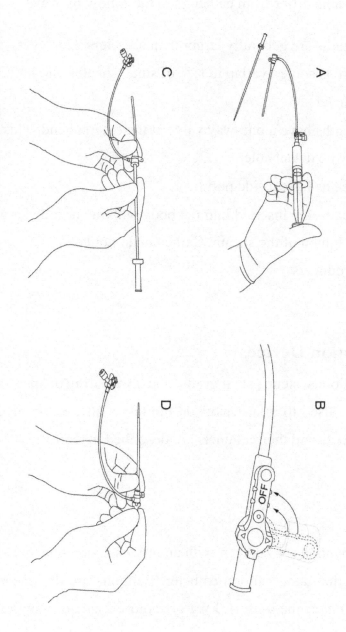

Figure 5.11 Sheath preparation

In general terms, catheters and sheaths go over wires and catheters go through sheaths. Though similar in their hollow design, sheaths differ from catheters in the following ways:

- Sheaths are generally larger than catheters. However, there is some overlap in size of small sheaths and large catheters.
- Sheaths have a one-way valve at the external end. This may be detachable.
- Sheaths have a side port.
- Sheaths are inserted into the body with the introducer in the lumen of the sheath. Catheters do not have introducers.

Intervention Devices

Balloons, stents, stent grafts, and a vast array of specialty devices are used to treat lesions at the target site. Some of the common tools and their adjuncts are described hereafter.

Balloon

A balloon is a catheter with an inflatable component at its tip-hence, the name balloon catheter. Balloons are designed in the coaxial/over the wire (OTW) or rapid exchange (monorail) configurations (figure 5.12). The basic design of the balloon consists of a hollow component that fits over a wire and a second compartment that is connected to the inflatable tip.

In the coaxial/OTW configuration, the device is mounted over and encloses the wire for the entirety of the length of the device (figure 5.12A). Balloons with this configuration have two ports—a port that conducts the wire, and a port for inflating and deflating the tip. The wire port is usually located at the external end of the device while the inflation port emanates at an angle from the long axis of the device. The minimum length of wire needed to convey an OTW device to the target site is a summation of the length of the device and the distance from the access site to the target site.

In the rapid exchange (monorail) configuration, the device is circumferential over the wire only for a segment of the length of the device (figure 5.12B). The wire emanates from the side of the device and the port at the external end of the device is used to inflate the balloon. The minimum length of wire needed to convey it to the target is a summation of the distance from the access site to the target site and the length of the device that encloses the wire. This is typically shorter than the length of wire needed in the OTW configuration.

The parts of a balloon are shown in figure 5.13. A request for a balloon includes its diameter, length, shaft length (working length), diameter of the wire that conducts it, and the size of the conducting sheath. Based on the characteristics of the surface of the balloon, they are generally classified as:

- Plain: Therapeutic effect delivered via radial force
- Drug coated: Has a medication coating which is applied to the target site at inflation
- Cutting/scoring: Modified surface to produce controlled cuts on the vessel wall

Example balloon diameters: 2.5mm, 3mm, 4mm, 6mm, 10mm

Example balloon lengths: 20mm, 40mm, 60mm, 120mm

Example shaft lengths (working length): 75cm, 80cm, 135cm

Example conducting wire diameters: 0.014in, 0.018in, 0.035in

Example conducting sheath diameters: 4Fr, 5Fr, 6Fr, 9Fr

For example, a request for a 4mm by 40mm balloon on an 80cm shaft implies a balloon that is 4mm in diameter and 40mm (4cm) in length. This balloon is mounted on a delivery device that is 80cm in length. This length can vary depending on the distance between the sites of access and therapeutic intervention.

The device packaging goes on to specify that the device should be conveyed on a wire no more than 0.018in in diameter and through a sheath that is at least 4Fr in diameter.

Preparation

-Flush the wire port with saline. Do not flush the inflation port as this will inflate the balloon and alter its insertion profile/size or it will prematurely disseminate the medication coating. It is recommended to avoid direct contact with the surface of a drug-eluting balloon. The manufacturers might provide a protective cover for this purpose. Otherwise, a dry piece of gauze placed over the surface as it is transferred onto the wire and into the body is helpful.

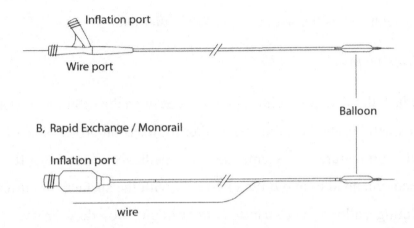

Figure 5.12 Balloons A: Coaxial/Over the wire configuration; B: Rapid exchange/Monorail configuration

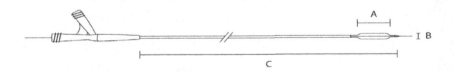

Figure 5.13 Parts of a balloon. A: Balloon length; B: Balloon diameter; C: Device shaft/working length

Balloons are inflated to specific diameters based on manufacturer's recommendations. The recommended pressures are contained on the insert provided in the balloon packaging (figure 5.14). This should be provided to the operator for reference prior to inflation. The nominal pressure is the pressure applied to the balloon to achieve its rated diameter. The burst pressure is the pressure below which there is a high certainty that the balloon will not burst. Inflating a balloon beyond the burst pressure is discouraged. The nominal and burst pressures are shown in different formats. In the format depicted in figure 5.14 A, the pressure (atmospheres) and diameter (mm) ratings for a specific balloon are shown on one table. In a different format, the pressure and associated diameters for several balloon diameters are shown on one table (figure 5.14 B). The ratings for each balloon vary based on size, type and manufacturer.

8.00mm balloon		
Pressure (atm)	Diameter	
8	-	
10	8.0	Nominal
12	8.1	
14	8.2	
16	8.3	
18	8.4	
20	8.5	Rated burst pressure
22	-	
24	-	

Figure 5.14 A The 8mm balloon depicted in this example achieves its nominal diameter of 8mm when a pressure of 10atm is applied. It is recommended not to exceed the burst pressure of 20 atm.

Balloon diameter (mm)	Inflation pressure (atm)								
	4	5	6	7	8	9	10	11	12
3.0	-	-	3.0	3.1	3.2	3.3	**BP**	-	-
4.0	-	-	4.0	4.1	4.2	4.3	**BP**		
5.0	-	-	5.0	5.1	5.2	5.3	**BP**		
6.0	-	6.0	6.1	6.2	**BP**				
7.0	-	7.0	7.1	7.2	**BP**				

Figure 5.14 B In this example, a 4mm balloon achieves its nominal diameter when a pressure of 6 atmospheres is applied. The burst pressure is 10atm. A 6mm balloon by the same manufacturer/class achieves its nominal diameter at 5atm and has a rated burst pressure of 8atm.

Stents

A stent is a hollow implant that is applied to the target site (figure 5.15). The basic stent design consists of a metal or metalloid lattice. Stents delivery systems may also be coaxial/OTW or rapid exchange (monorail) in configuration. The difference in design and considerations pertaining to conducting wire lengths described under the section on balloons also apply. Stents are generally classified as:

- Plain (bare metal) stent: Simple lattice
- Covered stent (stent graft): The lattice is covered with fabric thus making it impermeable to blood.
- Drug eluting stent: The stent is coated with medication

The tensile strength, radial force, and conformability can be modified to yield a wide variety of stents for various purposes. All stents can be expanded after deployment with a balloon. The term "balloon expandable stent" refers to a type of stent, which among other properties, is preloaded on a balloon and deployed via inflation of the balloon. Other stents are deployed through a variety of mechanisms depending on the manufacturer. These stents may or may not be further expanded with a balloon after deployment. A request for a stent includes the stent diameter, stent length, length of the shaft (working length), diameter of the wire that conducts the stent, and the size of the conducting sheath.

Example stent diameters: 3mm, 4mm, 6mm 10mm

Example stent lengths: 20mm, 28mm, 38mm, 40mm, 60mm, 120mm

Example shaft lengths (working length): 75cm, 80cm, 135cm

Example conducting wire diameters: 0.014in, 0.018in, 0.035in

Example conducting sheath diameters: 4Fr, 5Fr, 6Fr, 7Fr

A request for an 8mm by 40mm stent on a 135cm shaft implies a stent that is 8mm in diameter and 40mm in length, mounted on a delivery system that is 135cm in length. The device packaging specifies that the device should be conveyed on a 0.035in wire and through a sheath that is at least 6Fr in diameter.

Preparation

-Significant variability exists in the mechanisms by which stents are delivered and deployed. However, it is often necessary to flush the wire port.

-Balloon-mounted stents have a wire port and an inflation port. It is critical to flush the wire port but not the inflation port. Erroneous insufflation of the inflation port during preparation will prematurely deploy the stent. The wire port is usually at the external tip of the device while the inflation port emanates at an angle from the long axis of the device. Most manufacturers also label these ports for clarity.

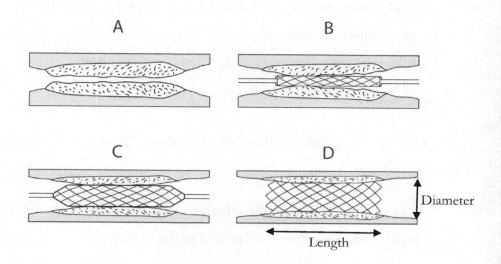

Figure 5.15 Stents. A: Lesion; B: Pre-deployed stent in position; C: Stent deployed; D: Device removed

Balloon Adjunct: Insufflation Device

This device is used to generate controlled inflation of a balloon or deployment of a balloon-mounted stent (figure 5.16). The insufflator is loaded with contrast (e.g., one-third or quarter strength contrast). The contrast in the insufflator/balloon allows visualization of the expanding balloon under fluoroscopy. Manual pressure generated by the operator is transmitted to the balloon through the fluid-filled chamber. The pressure applied is measured by the manometer. The manufacturer's guide on the recommended pressure range should be referenced on the package insert. Insufflators have a locking mechanism that allows the balloon to be locked in an inflated or deflated position. Large syringes can also be used to inflate balloons in large blood vessels. However, the pressure applied is not monitored.

Preparation

- Load the insufflator with contrast, without filling the chamber (figure 5.17).

- Leave some room in the chamber to allow application of negative pressure after it is attached to the balloon.

- Purge any excess air.

- Apply negative pressure to the insufflator after attachment to the inflation port. Tilt the insufflator such that the fluid fills the lower aspect of the contrast chamber and residual air within the balloon and conduction tract is displaced to the upper part of the contrast chamber prior to insufflation. This minimizes air artifact during inflation as well as the risk of air embolism in the rare event that the balloon ruptures while in use.

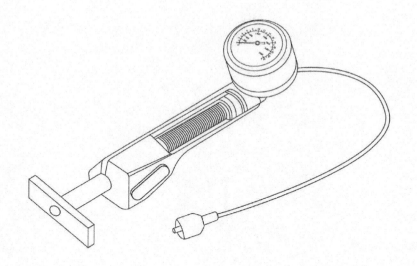

Figure 5.16 Insufflator

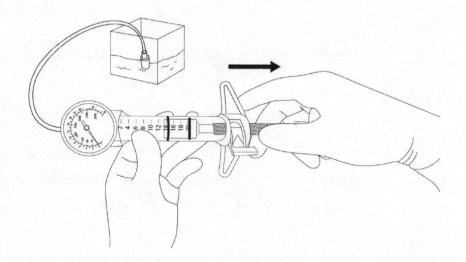

Figure 5.17 A Partially fill chamber with contrast (dilute)

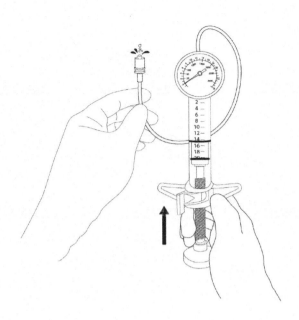

Figure 5.17 B Purge excess air

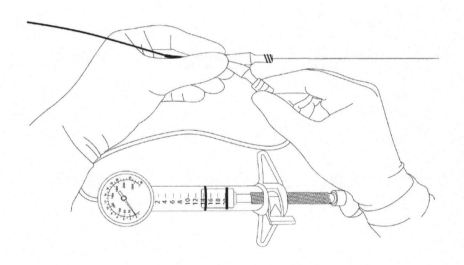

Figure 5.17 C Attach insufflator to insufflation port of device

Specialty Devices

A wide array of devices and implants exist for intervention in the cardiovascular system beyond those described in the preceding section. They include but are not limited to:

- Thrombectomy/embolectomy devices
- Thrombolytic devices
- Embolization devices
- Embolic protection devices
- Atherectomy devices
- Endograft fixation devices
- Snares
- Re-entry devices
- Ablation devices
- Fractional flow reserve devices
- Pressure transducing devices
- Atrial appendage closure devices
- Valves and clips

There is significant variability in their design, method of preparation, and deployment. These descriptions exceed the scope of this book. However, they can be found in the respective manufacturer's guides.

Contrast

Contrast agents are radiopaque fluids that are injected into the body in order to outline the anatomy under fluoroscopy. Contrast agents are also used to inflate balloons so their expansion can be visualized in real time. Some of the commonly used contrast agents are iodine-containing compounds and carbon dioxide gas. It is important to ask the operator what type and concentration of contrast is desired. Half-strength contrast contains equal parts of contrast and saline. Quarter-strength contrast contains one-part contrast and three-parts saline.

Syringe

Because different fluids or medications may be injected during the procedure, it is recommended to use color-coded or labelled syringes to keep track of the various fluid contents and to prevent erroneous injection. Do not completely fill the syringe with fluid and purge excess air (figure 5.18). The extra space in the chamber leaves room for the operator to apply negative pressure before injecting the contents of the syringe.

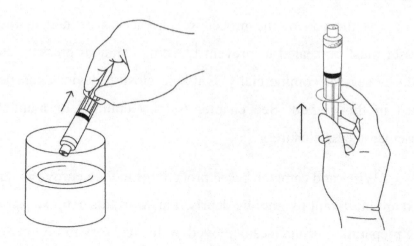

Figure 5.18 Loading a syringe. Partially load the syringe, and purge excess air. Thus, leaving space for negative pressure to be applied after attachment to device

Supplies

Scalpels, sutures, scissors, forceps, clamps, gauze, and radio opaque rulers are some of the common supplies that may be utilized for these procedures. The exact supplies needed depend on the procedure and are often provided in standardized packs or are readily accessible in the procedure rooms.

Closure Devices

At the end of the procedure, the access created in the vessel must be sealed to prevent bleeding. Manual pressure as well as several commercially available closure devices can be used in this regard. See chapter 6 for technique of manual vascular access closure.

Wire- and catheter-based procedures in the neurovascular bed are intolerant to embolic debris. This warrants extra steps in the preparation of devices deployed in this territory to minimize the risk of stroke. Additional steps taken to ensure that the devices are devoid of air or debris capable of embolizing into the brain may include inflating and deflating balloons and flushing or submerging the device tip in fluid prior to insertion. The type and extent of preparation vary by device type and should be communicated with the operator.

The steps for device preparation that we have described in this chapter are generic and in no way exhaustive. Preparatory steps vary by device and manufacturer. It is important to follow the manufacturer's recommended method of preparation.

Chapter 6

EXECUTION, COMMUNICATION AND SAFETY

Many aspects of wire- and catheter-based procedures are analogous to a choreographed dance. Actions are anticipated, and seamlessly accompanied by predictable reactions. The knowledge and preparatory steps described in the preceding chapters culminate in execution of the procedure. The goal of these procedures is to diagnose a problem or to treat a lesion. In some instances, the procedure commences with a diagnostic goal and evolves to achieve therapeutic objectives. The steps of the procedure depend on the type of procedure; in some instances, multiple approaches exist. A description of the steps for these procedures exceeds the scope of this text but some general concepts for their safe and successful execution are described below.

Personnel, equipment, and device preparation should conform to precautionary standards for asepsis (sterility) and radiation safety. These include:

- Covers for hair, eyes, nose, and mouth

- Precautions to minimize radiation exposure as outlined in Chapter 3
- Hand washing
- Sterile and fluid-resistant attire for all personnel within the sterile field: gowns, gloves
- Sterile preparation and draping of relevant patient parts
- Sterile draping of surfaces and equipment within the sterile field: Fluoroscopy machine, ultrasound probes and cords, operator controlled panels, radiation shields

The procedure should begin with a safety pause during which the identity of the patient and personnel, procedural side and site, objectives, equipment, allergies, and steps taken to mitigate infection are reviewed. It is good practice to encourage all personnel present to speak up at any point during the procedure if they notice any event that may compromise the safety of the patient or personnel.

Thereafter, the procedure progresses in a manner necessary to accomplish the diagnostic or therapeutic objective. The general idea involves the use of needles, wires, catheters, and sheaths to access the vascular system at one location and then to navigate the length, turns, and branches of the cardiovascular tree to reach the target for diagnosis or treatment (figure 6.1). Common sites for accessing the vascular system include radial, brachial, axillary, femoral, tibial and carotid locations. Depending on location, access may be percutaneous or open (via a cut down). Vascular access sites can also be classified as antegrade or retrograde in relation to the direction of blood flow. For example, femoral access with the needle and devices pointing cephalad is retrograde while, femoral access with needle and devices pointing caudad is antegrade. After vascular access is obtained, beginners and peri-procedural personnel may be required to assist with device retrieval, preparation, exchange, delivery, or deployment. Hence, the need to be familiar with the contents of this book.

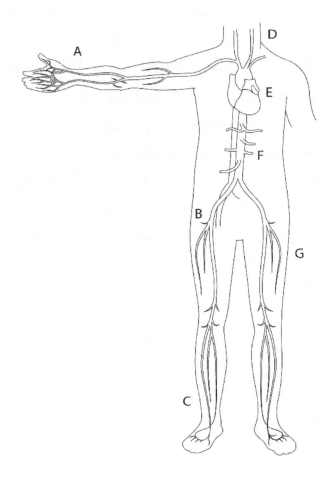

Figure 6.1 Access and intervention sites. The vascular system can be accessed at different locations such as the radial (A), femoral (B) and tibial (C) vessels for diagnostic or therapeutic interventions in other locations such as the carotid (D), coronary (E), visceral (F) or lower extremity (G) vascular beds.

Most procedures involve several device exchanges and the number of exchanges increases with procedure complexity. It is important to identify the components of the assembly that should move and components that should remain stationary when on- or off-loading a device. For example, when loading a catheter unto a wire, the catheter is the mobile component of the assembly, while the wire is static. This principle also applies when loading a sheath or any other device unto a wire. Conversely, when off-loading a device such as a catheter, balloon or stent delivery system, the device being off-loaded is the mobile component of the assembly, while the wire and sheath are held in place. Coordinated action by two persons may be required to efficiently and safely on- or off-load a device without disrupting the stationary component of the assembly. Stabilizing both hands on a rigid surface when on- or off-loading prevents loss of wire position.

.

Device On-loading

Prior to device on-loading, attention should be paid to the length of the shaft of the device (working length) relative to the length of wire available outside of the body. The length of wire outside the body should be greater than the device working length to ensure that the device can be on-loaded without losing position of the wire inside the body. The technique of device on-loading (pin and push) can be accomplished in four phases:

Phase 1: Loading the tip of the device unto the wire

Phase 2: Advancing the device over the wire until the external end of the wire exits the rear end of the device

Phase 3: Advancing the device until its leading end reaches the sheath/vessel access site

Phase 4: advancing the device within the sheath/body until the leading end reaches the target location

Phase 1: Loading the tip of the device unto the wire

Loading the tip of a device unto a wire or inserting a wire into a catheter can be straightforward or it can be the source of humorous jitter. The manual and visual coordination needed to load the tip of a device unto a wire can be enhanced by leveraging on the tactile and spatial properties of the finger pad and tip. This can be done by stabilizing the receiving device in a pinch grip between the pad of the index finger and the tip of the thumb (figure 6.2A). The secondary device is then inserted using the contralateral hand. This technique is often more efficient than connecting the devices in space (figure 6.2B). The device being advanced over the wire can also be preceded with moist gauze.

This clears any blood residue on the wire, lubricates it, and improves the efficiency of transfer (figure 6.3).

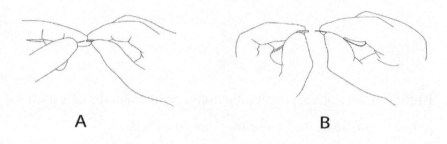

A   B

Figure 6.2 Loading devices unto a wire on the pulp of index finger (A) is often more efficient than loading in space (B)

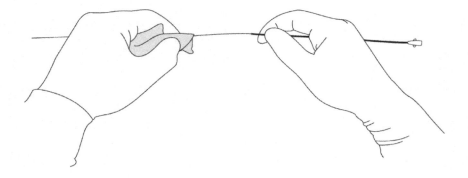

Figure 6.3 Device on-loading may be preceded with a moist gauze to lubricate and clear the wire of debris.

Phase 2: Advancing the device over the wire until the external end of the wire exits the rear end of the device

- Step 1: Pin the wire between the tip of the thumb and pulp of the index finger. This is done with the hand (hand 1) that is closer to the sheath/vascular access (figure 6.4). This maneuver keeps the wire stationary during the push phase.

- Step 2: With the second hand (hand 2), advance the leading end of the device over the wire until it reaches the position of hand 1(figures 6.5 and 6.6).
- Step 3: Move hand 1 to a new location on the wire away from the leading end of the device and closer to the sheath/vascular access site/the body (figure 6.7).

Hand 1 pins the wire at the new location to initiate another cycle of steps 1,2 and 3. These steps are repeated until the exterior end of the wire exits the rear end of the device (figure 6.8). Depending on the length of wire and device, it may be necessary to have a second person look out for the wire as it exits the rear end of the device and to communicate that this event has occurred. E.g "I have the wire" (after gaining manual control of the wire).

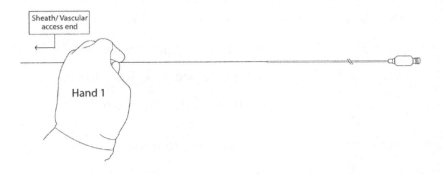

Figure 6.4 Pin the wire between the tip of the thumb and pulp of the index finger. This is done with the hand (hand 1) that is closer to the sheath/vascular access.

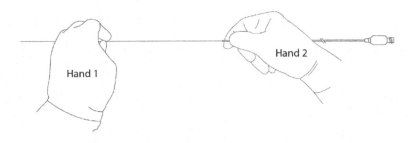

Figure 6.5 Grasp the leading end of the device.

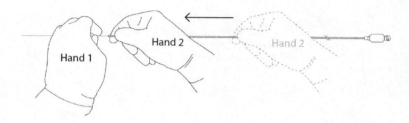

Figure 6.6 Advance (push) the leading end of the device over the wire until it reaches the position of hand 1

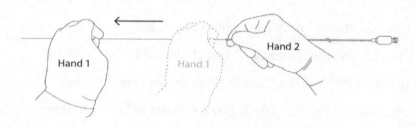

Figure 6.7 Move hand 1 to a new location on the wire away from the leading end of the device and closer to the sheath/vascular access site/the body.

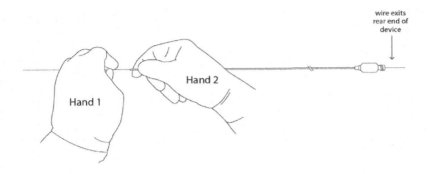

wire exits
rear end of
device

Hand 2

Hand 1

Figure 6.8 Repeat the sequence of pinning the wire and pushing the device over it until the external end of the wire exits the rear end of the device.

The distance between the hands 1 and 2, over which hand 2 travels to advance the device towards hand 1 should not be too long. Excess "travel" may cause bucking of the wire (figure 6.9). Conversely, the distance of travel should be long enough to accomplish efficient exchange. The appropriate distance varies with type of wire, size of device, friction between device and wire and experience. Caution is warranted when on-loading devices with special tips. These include tips with medication coating or components that should not be touched or compressed. Adherence to the manufacturer recommendations is advised.

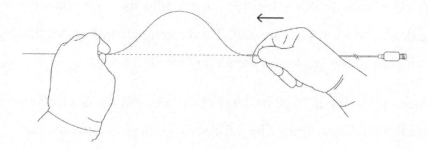

Figure 6.9 The distance of travel should not be too long to prevent bucking of the wire during the push step.

Phase 3: Advancing the wire until the leading end reaches the sheath

In a one-person setup:

- Step 1: Relocate hand 2 to the segment of wire distal to exterior end of the device. Pin the wire at this location (figure 6.10).
- Step 2: with hand 1, slide the device over the wire rail until the leading end reaches the hub of the sheath/access point (figure 6.10).

This phase can also be accomplished with the help of an assistant. This is especially helpful when working with a long device or wire. In this setup, person two pins the wire distal to the device to form the wire-rail. Thereafter, person 1 slides the device along the rail to the sheath and into the body.

When the device is large or the friction between the device and wire is significant. It may be necessary for person 1 to advance the device in several steps as opposed to one single motion. In this case, person 2 should follow the rear end of the device as it is advanced and pin the wire just distal to this end. Person 2 should not let go of the wire when the device been advanced. Otherwise, the wire position is lost. A safe approach is to use both hands to pin the wire. To accomplish this, one hand maintains control of the wire while the other hand moves closer to the rear end of the advancing device. As such wire control is not compromised at any instant.

It is possible to repeat the steps in phase 2 until the leading end of the device reaches the hub of the sheath/vessel access point. However, it is more efficient to slide the device over the wire after the segment of wire distal to the device is pinned.

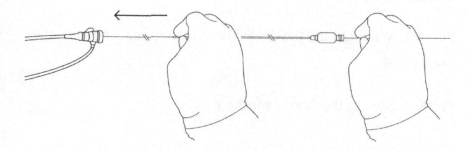

Figure 6.10 Pin the wire distal to the device and slide the device along the wire rail until the leading end reaches the hub of the sheath/access point.

Phase 4: Advancing the device within the sheath/body until the leading end reaches the target location.

With the wire rail maintained either by hand 2 or person 2. The device is advanced in the sheath and body until the leading end reaches the target location. This phase is commonly accomplished under fluoroscopic guidance. The aforementioned steps become smooth and automatic practice and experience.

Device Off-loading

The pin and pull technique of device off-loading can be accomplished in 2 phases.

Phase 1: Withdrawing the device until the internal end exits the sheath/body

Phase 2: Sliding the device off the wire.

Phase 1: Withdrawing the device until the internal end exits the sheath/body

- Step 1: Person 1 stabilizes the sheath so that it does not pull out of the patient as the device is withdrawn (Figure 6.11). If the device being withdrawn is the vascular access sheath, then person 1 prepares to manually control the access site (by compression) until control of the vascular access site is regained with another device.

The following steps are executed by person 2

- Step 2: Pin the wire with the hand further away from the device (hand 1). This stabilizes the wire so it does not move during the pull phase (figure 6.11).

- Step 3: with hand 2, pull the device over the wire until the hub reaches the position of hand 1 on the wire (figure 6.11).
- Step 4: Relocate hand 1 to a position away from the device on the wire and pin the wire at this location (figure 6.12).

This sequence of pinning the wire and pulling the device over it (pin & pull technique) is repeated (figures 6.13 & 6.14) until the inner end of the device exits the sheath (figure 6.15). At this point, person 1 pins the wire at this location and communicates that the device has exited the sheath. E.g "I have the wire" (after gaining manual control of the wire).

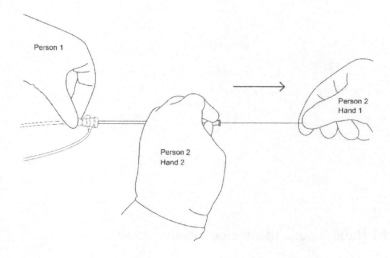

Figure 6.11 Person 1 holds the sheath. Person 2-hand 1 pins the wire. Person 2-hand 2 pulls the device

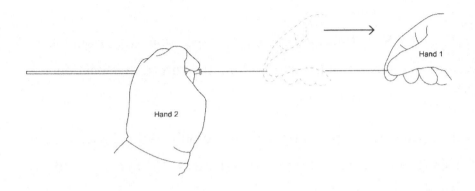

Figure 6.12 Hand 1 moves to a new location on the wire and pins the wire at that location

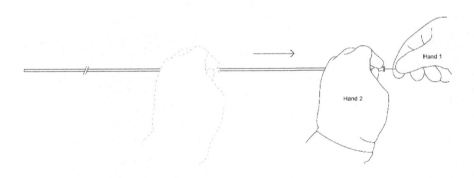

Figure 6.13 Hand 2 pulls the device towards hand 1

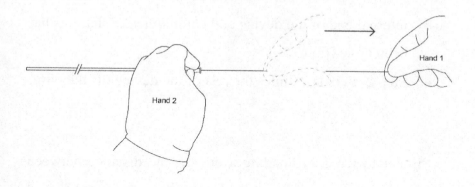

Figure 6.14 Hand 1 moves to a new location on the wire and pins the wire at that location

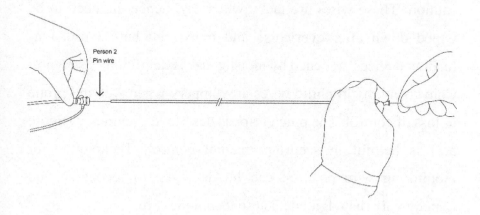

Figure 6.15 Person 1 pins the wire between sheath and end of device and communicates that this has been done.

Phase 2: Sliding the device off the wire.

- Step 1: Person 1 pins the wire between the sheath and the internal end of the device and communicates that this has been done (figure 6.15).
- Step 2: Person 2 slides the rest of the device off the wire.

Similar to when on-loading a device, the distance between both hands (over which the pull phase will be executed) should be short to prevent the wire from bucking but long enough for efficient off-loading. The balance of efficiency and safety is attained with practice and experience.

Device exchanges over hydrophilic wires warrant extra caution. These wires are tacky when dry, hence the need to be wiped down after every use and moistened before use. On-loading devices preceded by moist gauze is helpful in this regard. Conversely, hydrophilic wires are slippery when wet and prone to loss of control. The pinch grip, as described previously (figure 5.3) is helpful in securing manual control. Techniques for monitoring wire position can be deployed to recognize and remedy wire dislodgment. These techniques are:

- Intermittent confirmation of the position of the internal end of the wire under fluoroscopy as the device exchange proceeds.

- Marking and monitoring the external end of the wire on a stationary surface. To do this, the position of the external end of the wire is marked on the table with a marker or object prior to device exchange. The position of the external end of the wire is monitored relative to this mark as the exchange is carried out. Of note, the internal end of the wire can still be dislodged if the wire bucks anywhere between the internal and external ends, hence the need to meticulously maintain rigid wire position.

Loss of Access

After access into the vascular system and across the target has been obtained, it is important to maintain it. Loss of access due to dislodgement of wire, catheter, or sheath can be a source of frustration for several reasons:

- Vascular access and traversal of the cardiovascular tree to the target can be time consuming. Loss of access calls for repeat maneuvers that lengthen the duration of the procedure.

- Uncontrolled forward dislodgement carries the risk of perforation, dissection, and embolization.
- Maneuvers to regain access increase the risk of embolization, dissection, and other complications.
- Loss of access at the vascular entry site leads to bleeding.
- It may be impossible to regain access, thus compromising the success of the procedure.

A setup that prioritizes organization, elimination of the effect of gravity on devices, communication, and meticulous device exchange is key to avoiding loss of access and the aforementioned risks.

- Avoid back table clutter by organizing devices between uses in an easily retrievable manner. Discard packages and devices that are **certain not to be reused**.
- Use table extensions along the axis of access to provide support to devices and to prevent inadvertent motion under the influence of gravity (figure 6.16).
- Communicate clearly.
- Exchange devices meticulously.

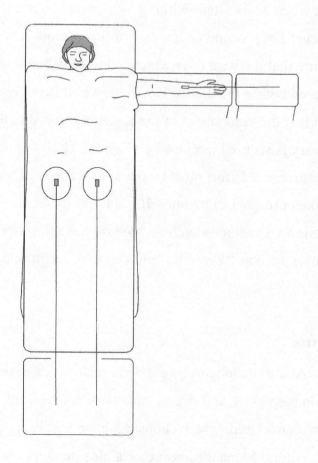

Figure 6.16 Table extensions along the axis of access can stabilize devices, provide a supporting surface for exchanges and minimize dislodgement and loss of access

One of the most common scenarios leading to loss of access occurs when an assistant withdraws a device over a wire that is not secured in position (pinned). For this reason, it is imperative to ensure that the wire over which a device is being withdrawn is secured before the device is withdrawn. It is not enough to expect that the component of the assembly that should be stationary is secured in place by someone else. Assumptions can be catastrophic! Effort must be made to secure the stationary component (e.g wire) by oneself or clarify that a team member has done so. Questions such as "do you have the wire?" and responses such as "Yes, I do" are key to preventing mishaps.

Closure

Anatomic location, vessel characteristics, size of the hole made in the vessel, and degree of anticoagulation are some of the factors considered when choosing how to close the vascular access points. Manual pressure or a closure device may be used to seal the hole made in the vessel. Descriptions of the various closure devices exceeds the scope of this text. However, details of their description, preparation, and deployment are provided by the manufacturers.

Manual pressure is a reliable method of access site closure. The goal is to apply pressure over the hole in the vessel long enough to allow a clot to seal it and to allow further healing over time. It is important to understand the anatomic relationships at the access site in order to effectively seal the hole and prevent complications. When obtaining vascular access, the needle is directed at an angle and passes through the skin and subcutaneous tissue before piercing the vessel (Figure 6.17). The distance of the hole in the vessel from the skin puncture in the horizontal plane depends on the angle of needle entry and depth of subcutaneous tissue. The focus of vascular access closure should be directed at sealing the hole in the vessel. Digital pressure applied a centimeter or two proximal to the skin puncture is usually sufficient (Figure 6.18).

The venous system is less pressurized than the arterial system, so the duration and amount of pressure needed to seal a venous puncture is less than that needed to seal an arterial puncture. The duration of manual pressure should be discussed with the operator. Improper technique or inadequate duration of manual closure can lead to potentially life-threatening complications such as bleeding and formation of pseudo aneurysms.

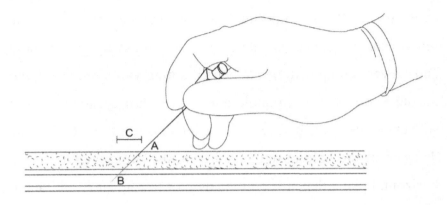

Figure 6.17 Vascular access. A: skin puncture site, B: vessel puncture site, C: distance between skin and vessel puncture sites in horizontal plane.

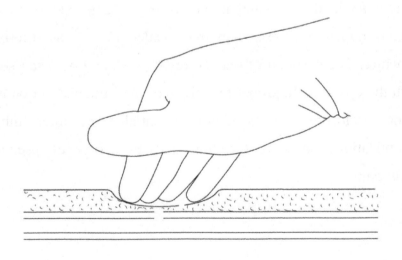

Figure 6.18 Closure of vascular access site by manual pressure

Communication

The teamwork required to safely, efficiently, and successfully complete a procedure is largely dependent on effective communication. A two-step process of request and verbal read back prior to execution of an action is recommended to confirm common understanding. This process is especially important when it involves requests to pull tools or devices out from the body, because misunderstanding these requests can result in loss of access. Actions on the wire-device assembly are often accompanied by a concomitant reaction. Communication fosters the synchrony of actions while asynchrony can result in undesirable loss of access, maldeployment, injury, or other mishaps. Inaction may be warranted at other times during the procedure. These should be communicated clearly and clarified as needed. The need for robust communication cannot be over emphasized. Some statements commonly made during the procedure include:

"I have the wire"

"I am holding onto/pinning the wire"

"I am letting go of the wire"

"You said pull out the wire, correct?"

"I am holding the sheath"

"I am pulling out the catheter"

"I am pulling the sheath"

"Do you have the wire?"

Communication is a crucial part of patient experience and satisfaction. While the procedure and the environment might be familiar to the personnel, they are unfamiliar to the patient. An awake patient should be told what is going on, and personnel should inquire and address anxiety, pain, or other stimuli. It is important to communicate professionally at all times. Patients can sense the atmosphere in the procedure room, be it cordial or otherwise; this can affect their overall satisfaction. Patients' recollection of unprofessional conduct or communication during a procedure can erode the impact of an otherwise successful procedure. It is possible to hear, retain, and recollect conversations even when sedated.

Safety

The safety of the patient and personnel is top priority. Knowledge and skill are key elements of procedural safety. It is important for personnel to speak up when they notice an impending, occurring, or past event that constitutes a safety risk to the patient or personnel. Accordingly, it is important to promote a culture in which personnel can speak freely about safety concerns and express ideas for quality improvement. Instances when it is mandatory to speak up include, but are not limited to, a break in sterile technique or radiation protection.

Complications can occur and the overall impact of a complication is dependent on prompt recognition and address. Bleeding, hematoma, and loss of distal extremity arterial signals/pulses are some of the complications that can be recognized by any member of the team. Prompt escalation and intervention are key to limiting their impact.

Common units of measurement and examples of needles, wires, catheters, sheaths, balloons and stents

Needles

Diameter *(Gauge): 18Ga, 21Ga

Wires

Diameter (inches): 0.010, 0.014, 0.018, 0.035 inches...

Length (centimeters): 45cm, 150cm, 180cm, 260cm, 300cm...

Catheters

Diameter **(French): 3 Fr, 4Fr, 5Fr, 8Fr...

Length (centimeters): 65cm, 100cm, 125cm...

Sheaths

Diameters (French): 4fr, 5Fr, 6Fr, 12Fr...

Length (centimeters): 10cm, 40cm, 70cm...

Balloons

Diameter (millimeters): 3mm, 4mm, 6mm…

Length (millimeters): 20mm, 40mm, 60mm…

    ***(centimeters): 2cm, 4cm, 6cm…

Shaft length (centimeters): 75cm, 80cm, 125cm, 135cm…

Stents

Diameter (millimeters): 3mm, 4mm, 6mm…

Length (millimeters): 20mm, 40mm, 60mm…

    **(centimeters): 2cm, 4cm, 6cm…

Shaft length (centimeters): 75cm, 80cm, 125cm, 135cm…

*In the gauge measurement system, diameter decreases with increasing gauge number. Hence, the 21Ga needle has a smaller diameter than the 18Ga needle.

**In the French measurement system, diameter increases with increase in French number.

***The length of a balloon or stent may be described in cm. Hence, the metric conversion between mm and cm should be borne in mind.

Made in the USA
Coppell, TX
31 July 2023

19794807R00059